INNER EAR INFECTIONS CURE

Natural Home Remedies for Ear Infections, Treatment and Prevention

By

Kim Hilton

INNER EAR INFECTIONS CURE

First edition. July, 2018.

Copyright © 2018 Kim Hilton

Written by Kim Hilton

Books by The Same Author

- <u>Boost Your Energy Levels: 60 Natural Ways to Get Rid of Fatigue, Dizziness, Weakness, And Lack of Motivation</u>

- <u>How to Get Rid Of Stretch Marks Naturally</u>

- <u>How to Break Sugar Cravings with Nutritional Supplements:</u> Healthy and Natural Alternatives

- <u>The Anti-Anxiety Cookbook:</u> Nutritional Plan to Cure Depression and Anxiety (Stress Relief and Mental Health Cookpot)

- <u>Eating Disorder Recovery Workbook:</u> How to Recover from

Eating Disorder On Your Own (Anorexia, Bulimia Nervosa, And Binge Eating)

- <u>100 Health Hacks Nobody Ever Told You:</u> **Natural Tips and Tricks for Enhanced and Prudent Well-Being**

- <u>How to Lower Blood Pressure Naturally & Quickly: Powerful Tricks to Deal with Hypertension Using Supplements and Other Natural Remedies</u>

- <u>Reverse Type 2 Diabetes: How to Control and Prevent Diabetes Naturally</u>

- <u>Urinary Tract Infection Treatment: Home Remedies for Urinary Tract Infections and Prevention Methods</u>

- <u>Natural Treatments for Yeast Infection: How to Cure a Yeast Infection Using Home Remedies</u>
- <u>Itchy Skin Solution: Effective Home Remedies to Get Rid of Dry, Itchy Skin</u>
- <u>Top 30 Cancer-Fighting Foods: Diets and Nutritional Meal Plans to Manage, Overcome, and Prevent Cancer</u>
- <u>Home Remedies for Toothache: Natural Ways to Relieve Severe Toothache and Gum Pain</u>

Table of Contents

Introduction

Ear infection is a very common health challenge that occurs in both kids and adults. It can be induced by bacteria, viruses and in rare cases, yeast. Studies have shown that ear infection occurs both in humans and pets, such as dogs.

Ear infections also occurs when one of your Eustachian tube becomes blocked or swollen, this leads to fluid retention in the middle ear.

The ears are important and complicated organs of the body, they are the organs responsible for hearing and they also help with balance. The severe pain experienced in ear infections is caused by accumulation of fluid in the middle ear and inflammation.

Ear infections in children are not serious and they clear on their own without any help, but ear infections in adults should not be taken lightly because they are usually signs of a serious medical problem.

Ear infections can be acute or chronic; Acute infections heal fast but they can be very painful. Chronic infections linger or they keep recurring. If left untreated, they can cause permanent damage to the inner and middle ear.

Types of Ear Infections

Ear infections are basically classified according to the part of the ear infected. Practically, the following are the know types of ear infection:

1. Outer ear infections (or otitis externa) which is also known as "swimmer's ear" is caused by bacterial skin tissues covering the ear canal, it is caused by immersion in water, letting water enter your ear when bathing, and putting things in your ear canal to remove earwax. It usually starts like an itchy rash.

2. "Middle Ear Infections (also called otitis media) is an infection that occurs behind the ear drum." It is characterized by pus trapped in the middle ear space of the facial bone causing the eardrum to bulge.

Middle ear infections usually occur with an infection of the upper respiratory tract and that is why symptoms of runny nose, sore throat, and sinus pressure are usually felt in middle ear infections.

Infections of the middle and outer ear are the most common ear infections.

3. Inner ear infections are primarily caused by viral infection even though it is mostly uncommon. This type of ear infection is characterized by inflammation of the structures which aid balance and earing.

Causes of Ear Infections

The common causes of inner ear infection are the harmful microorganism such as fungus, viruses and bacteria. The severity and duration depends on the method of infection.

People with compromised immune system and chronic diseases have the highest risk of inner ear infections.

Inflammation or blockage of the Eustachian tubes can also cause ear infections, factors that can cause this blockage or inflammation are smoking, allergies (know your triggers and avoid them), changes in air pressure, colds, infected adenoids, excess mucus and sinus infections.

Viruses are the main causes of inner ear infections. A less common cause of an inner ear infection is bacteria. Infections of the inner ear last longer than those of the middle and outer ear.

Inner Ear Infections

The inner ear connects the ear to the brain and it contains tubes and sacs filled with tubes and they are called labyrinth. The cochlea transmits sound signals to the brain thus helping with hearing while the vestibular organs help with balance by giving the brain information about head movement.

Infections of the inner ears are often caused by irritation or inflammation of the labyrinth, this is the part of the ear that aids hearing and balance. Difficulty hearing is more common in inner ear infections than middle or outer ear infections. Another name for infection of the inner ear is Labyrinthitis.

Some health experts argue that this is case of inflammation and may not actually be a true infection. In most cases, inner ear infections are caused by inflammation and microbial infections (true infections) are responsible for very few cases.

Viruses are mostly responsible for this infection and bacteria can cause this in few cases, inner ear infections are not contagious but the germs that cause them are. Viruses that can lead to inner ear infections are the polio virus, influenza virus, Epstein-Barr virus and herpes virus.

Prompt and proper treatment eliminates this infection in at most two weeks, this prevents hearing loss or permanent damage to the infected ear. Chronic infections of the ears can last up to 6 weeks.

Serious injury and trauma to the ear can also cause internal ear swelling and trauma and the pain depends on the severity of the injury.

Autoimmune conditions and harmful substances like some medications, illegal drugs and alcohol and other toxic substances can cause inflammation in the inner ear. Substances that are dangerous to the inner ear are known as ototoxic.

Some cases of inner ear infections result to permanent loss of hearing or partial hearing loss, and it also cause damage to the vestibular systems, the part of the ear controlling balance.

Symptoms specific to inner ear infections are sudden dizziness, tinnitus (ringing of the ears), vertigo, vomiting, nausea, and balance disruption. Inner ear infections could also be a symptom of meningitis.

Symptoms of Inner Ear Infections

The symptoms start at the beginning of the infection and are more severe at the beginning, symptoms are:

- A painful feeling inside the ear

- Discomforts inside the ear

- Scaly skin inside and the areas around the ear

- A high body temperature

- Itching inside the ear and outside

- Irritation and inflammation inside and the areas around the ear.

- Feeling sick

- Mild headache

- The affected ear becomes tender

- Feeling full inside the ear or a feeling of pressure inside and the areas around the ear

- Blurred or double vision or other changes in vision

- Difficulty walking or having balance

- Nausea and vomiting

- A spinning sensation

- Discharge or fluid coming out of the ear

- Fatigue and weaknesses

- Tinnitus

- Difficulty hearing or hearing loss

Symptoms in children and little babies are:

- Loss of balance

- Constantly rubbing their ear or pulling it

- Loss of appetite

- Inability to hear and they won't react to sounds

- Irritability and restlessness

Natural Treatments for Inner Ear Infections

Mullein

The leaves and flowers of this herb and its essential oil are one of the best and most effective natural remedies for earaches and infections. You can make use of pure mullein tinctures as eardrops or you can use mullein tinctures that have been combined with other herbs.

It is a natural anesthetic and it fights germs also. It is even used to treat ear infections in dogs too because of its potency.

Ginger

Ginger is a natural pain killer and it contains powerful anti-inflammatory compounds which makes it effective in treating all kinds of ear infections.

Crush fresh ginger root and extract the juice, apply it around the pinnacle and outer ear canal and not directly inside the ear. You can warm fresh ginger root in olive oil or coconut oil, strain it and apply it around the ear also but nit inside.

This will penetrate and heal the root cause of the infection and ache. You can also drink ginger tea many times daily or chew on fresh ginger root.

Vitamin D

Vitamin D fortifies the immune system and studies have confirmed its potency in curing ear infections. Increases exposure to mild sunlight and high intake of vitamin D rich foods like eggs and organic poultry are natural ways to boost the levels of vitamin D in your body and, this, in turn, will prevent and treat ear infections.

Vitamin D supplements are also available, meet a doctor to prescribe one for you.

Compresses

Cold or warm compresses help to relieve ear pains and aches and this remedy is safe for both adults and little children. One material which is important for the compress is ice packs, followed by damp clothes. Wrapping the ice pack in the clothing should be a kick-start for the whole process.

Choose the temperature you want, either hot or cold and place the compress over the infected ear. An effective way to get rid of pain is to alternate between hot and cold after ten minutes.

Breast milk

Breast milk help little babies develop a strong immune system and this remedy is effective for new born babies whose immune system is still developing, because finding a natural remedy suitable for them is difficult.

Breast milk is the best cure in this stage, breast milk is a powerful remedy and this is one reason why doctors recommend breastfeeding babies for one year.

Breast milk contains antibodies made completely by the mother of the baby, these will speed up healing and fight the infection. By breast feeding the baby, you are also boosting your child's immune system and kick starting it to get rid of the infection.

Putting drops of breast milk in your baby's ear will fight inflammation and relieve other symptoms of ear infections. It reduces swellings and enhances healing.

You can also rub breast milk around the ears and this remedy is surprisingly beneficial for adults also. Breast milk can also be used on minor injuries and wounds and even eye infections.

Castor Oil

This oil is loaded with antimicrobial and antiseptic compounds, it kills bacteria, fungi and any harmful germs that cause ear infections. Daily use of this oil kills all harmful germs in the ear.

Use warm oil so that the heat will soothe the skin in the inner ear and dissolve hardened ear wax. This is one of the best home remedies for ear pains and infections.

Slightly heat castor oil and put few drops inside the infected ear. Do this at night before going to bed. Put a cotton ball to prevent the oil from draining out and you should sleep with the infected ear facing upwards.

The first thing to do in the morning is to remove the cotton ball and wipe out every residue or oily substance in the ear, then you can rinse it with clean or mild soap water.

Garlic

This herb has pain relieving properties and it is a strong natural antibiotic which can fight the germs responsible for ear infections. Studies have confirmed that eardrops containing garlic and other herbal ingredients are as effective as OTC eardrops.

Get fresh garlic and crush them, soak them in either extra virgin olive oil or sesame oil for several minutes. Strain the solution to separate the crushed garlic and apply this oil inside your ear canals. Do this many times daily.

Apple Cider Vinegar

This is an excellent remedy for ear infections and pain, it prevents fungi from growing in the ear and its antimicrobial and antiseptic properties treats infections of the ear caused by microbes and germs.

It contains acids that kills off these harmful germs and eliminates bad substances accumulated in the ear. It fights inflammation and also boosts the immune system because it contains important nutrients.

You can make use of white vinegar but apple cider vinegar is more effective. Dilute it with water before putting it directly into the ear to prevent discomforts.

Or you soak a cotton ball in diluted and organic ACV and put it in your ear like an ear plug. Leave it in your ear for five minutes before taking it out. You can also massage your outer ear and its surrounding with diluted vinegar.

Gargling with apple cider vinegar is also helpful because the ears, nose and throat are connected via passages and this will help the liquid go up into your Eustachian tube and therefore works in getting rid of the main cause of the impairment.

Tea Tree Essential Oil

This essential is packed full with antimicrobial and antiseptic properties, it can be dropped in the ear to cure infections, inflammation, pain, irritations, and other symptoms. To avoid sensitivity, dilute this essential oil with extra virgin olive oil.

Salt

The use of salt according to studies have proven to be among the best natural and at home ways to treat inner ear infection. Ear drainage, which is important can be done easily using salt. Heated salt draws out fluids from the infected ear and it also relieves inflammation, pains and swellings.

You can make use of either salt or rice. Heat a cup of salt or a cup of rice over mild heat for five minutes, pour the hot salt or rice on a clean cloth. Use a knot or a rubber band to tie the open end and allow it to get warm.

"When it is warm, lay down and place this warm cloth against the infected ear for ten minutes. Do this daily." The heat and healing reaction of the salt will help drain the fluid. Symptoms are usually relieved once the fluids are completely drained out.

Hydrogen peroxide

For many years, this humble liquid has been used as to relieve earaches naturally. Several drops of hydrogen peroxide are dropped into the infected ear and left to sit in the ear for several minutes before being drained out.

After the whole proves you can rinse the ear with distilled and clean water. It is highly recommended to repeat this 3 times daily.

Mango Leaves

Mango leaves are effective in treating ear infection and they offer a quick relieve from earaches and pains. Get a good quantity of fresh and tender mango leaves and crush them so that you can get the juice.

Warm the juice with mild heat and put few drops of the warm juice into your ears making use of a dropper. This will give you instant relief from the pain.

This should be done three times daily to give you full relief from the pain and to also treat ear infections because mango leaves contain antimicrobial and antiseptic compounds.

Olive Oil

Warm olive oil is an effective folk remedy for ear infection and ear ache. It is safe and effective, it fights germs because pure virgin olive oil contains antimicrobial and antimicrobial properties.

To avoid burning your eardrum, use olive that is as warm as your body temperature. You can use a thermometer to be very sure.

Holy Basil

The leaves of this wonderful herb are loaded with antioxidants and therapeutic compounds and it also has a strong antibacterial, and antimicrobial property.

Pick fresh basil leaves and crush them to aid the extraction of the juice. Apply this juice on the infected and around it, but do this carefully to prevent the juice from entering inside the ear canal.

You can also use basil essential oil, dilute it with coconut oil or olive oil in equal amounts. Soak a cotton wool in the mixture and use to clean inside and around the ears, do it gently and also clean the outside of the ears.

Probiotics

This help to fortify the defense system and get rid of harmful microbes. It is even used in pediatric ear infections, you can get probiotics by eating fermented foods like cultured yogurt, coconut kefir, Kombucha and kimchi.

They are available in the form of supplements and capsules, regular intake of probiotics in your diet prevents ear infections from happening in the first place. Probiotics are healthy strains of bacteria that fight off harmful germs that can cause ear infections.

Coconut oil

The healthy fatty acids present in coconut oil contains antimicrobial properties, it also fights inflammation and relieves pain because it contains analgesic compounds.

Pour few drops of coconut oil into the infected ear and place a cotton ball in the ear so that the oil won't spill or leak out. Open and close your jaws few times, this will allow the oil go into all corners of the ear canal.

Leave the cotton wool in your ears for 20 minutes, do this two times daily.

Neck Exercises

Exercises can relieve ear pain caused by pressure in canal. Neck rotation exercises are beneficial, you can meet a physiotherapist to help you with some exercises and you can try the following in the comfort of your home.

- Sit straight and make sure that your both feet are flat on the ground

- Rotate your head and neck slowly to the right side until your head is parallel to your left shoulder

- Elevate your shoulders like you are trying to cover your ears with them

- These movements should be made slowly, stretch and hold gently at the count of 5 and then relax.

- Repeat this many times daily.

Proper Sleep Position

A bad sleeping position can aggravate the pain of ear infections while a good sleep position can relieve it. When sleeping, the infected ear should be elevated and not faced down on the pillow.

Use extra pillows to elevate your head and this will also help to drain the ears faster.

Naturopathic Eardrops

These eardrops are made from herbs and other natural extract, meet a doctor or a naturopath to prescribe one for you. There are as effective as the eardrops bought over-the-counter.

Chiropractic Adjustments

Chiropractic adjustments can also soothe ear pain. Misalignment in the spine can affect overall health and impair healing, studies have proven that there is a strong relationship between chiropractic adjustments and relieving ear infections in little children also.

Spinal re-alignment and manipulations relax the muscles that surround the Eustachian tubes thereby allowing pus and other fluid collected to drain. It also revamps the overall functions of the nervous system thus boosting the general health of the body.

How to Prevent Inner Ear Infections

It is not guaranteed that you can prevent inner ear infections because it is caused by colds and flu but there are steps you can take to reduce the risk of this infection.

• Stay away from smoky environment and don't let children stay in smoky environment.

• Don't smoke or quit smoking because this unhealthy habit increases the risk and frequency of respiratory infections and ear infections by damaging the delicate tissues of the body and it also damages the defense system.

•   Wash your hands regularly to prevent taking germs to your ear

•   Avoid putting your fingers or objects in your ear, they might be contaminated.

•   Avoid second-hand smoke

•   Breastfeed infants properly

When to see a Doctor

This is usually a mild infection and it clears off on its own in three days but if you feel or start experiencing any of the symptoms or conditions, and when it persists in the body, please visit a nearest health professional or doctor immediately.

- If the infection lasts more than one week

- A very high body temperature

- A chronic illness or long-term medical condition like heart disease, kidney problem, neurological problem, lung diseases, or diabetes.

- Feeling hot and shivery

- Swelling around the ear

- Change in hearing or inability to hear

- Fluid oozing out of the ear

- A weak or suppressed immune system

- Dizziness

- A severe sore throat

- Recurring ear infections

Risks of Chronic Ear Infections

When you have chronic ear infections and it is not properly treated or it re-occurs often, it raises the risks for the following health complications.

- A damaged or ruptured eardrum

- Loss of hearing or deafness

- Meningitis, a bacterial infection that covers the membranes of the spinal cord and brain

- Language or speech delay in children

- Mastoiditis, an infection that occurs in the mastoid bone located in the skull.

Books by The Same Author

- <u>Boost Your Energy Levels: 60 Natural Ways to Get Rid of Fatigue, Dizziness, Weakness, And Lack of Motivation</u>

- <u>How to Get Rid Of Stretch Marks Naturally</u>

- <u>How to Break Sugar Cravings with Nutritional Supplements:</u> Healthy and Natural Alternatives

- <u>The Anti-Anxiety Cookbook:</u> Nutritional Plan to Cure Depression and Anxiety (Stress Relief and Mental Health Cookpot)

- <u>Eating Disorder Recovery Workbook:</u> How to Recover from Eating Disorder On Your Own (Anorexia, Bulimia Nervosa, And Binge Eating)

- <u>100 Health Hacks Nobody Ever Told You:</u> Natural Tips and Tricks for Enhanced and Prudent Well-Being

- <u>How to Lower Blood Pressure Naturally & Quickly: Powerful Tricks to Deal with Hypertension Using Supplements and Other Natural Remedies</u>

- <u>Reverse Type 2 Diabetes: How to Control and Prevent Diabetes Naturally</u>

- <u>Urinary Tract Infection Treatment: Home Remedies for Urinary Tract Infections and Prevention Methods</u>

- <u>Natural Treatments for Yeast Infection: How to Cure a Yeast Infection Using Home Remedies</u>

- <u>Itchy Skin Solution: Effective Home Remedies to Get Rid of Dry, Itchy Skin</u>

- <u>Top 30 Cancer-Fighting Foods: Diets and Nutritional Meal Plans to Manage, Overcome, and Prevent Cancer</u>

- <u>Home Remedies for Toothache: Natural Ways to Relieve Severe Toothache and Gum Pain</u>